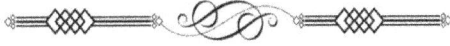

A Matter of The Heart

My Unexpected Journey with Diabetes

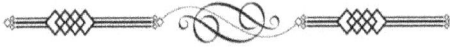

Mark D. Brezzell MS CP

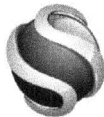

ASA PUBLISHING CORPORATION
AN INNOVATIVE OUTSOURCE BOOK PUBLISHING HYBRID

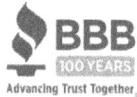

BBB
100 YEARS
Advancing Trust Together℠

ASA Publishing Corporation
An Accredited Hybrid Publishing House with the BBB
www.asapublishingcorporation.com
1285 N. Telegraph Rd., PMB 351, Monroe, Michigan 48162

This book was published in the United States of America.
Great State of Michigan

DEDICATION

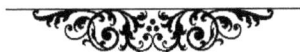

This book is dedicated to all those who battle with diabetes every day. Your strength, resilience, and determination are an inspiration to us all. May our shared experiences bring hope, understanding, and a sense of community to everyone affected by this condition.

ACKNOWLEDGMENT

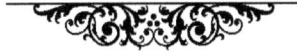

I am delighted to extend my deepest gratitude to my loving wife, Cleo. Your unwavering love and support have been my anchor throughout this journey. Your strength and encouragement have been invaluable, and I am forever grateful to have you in my life.

A heartfelt thank you to Dr. Kim Logan-Nowlin for encouraging me to share my story, and Dr. David Williams's critical review is unprecedented. Your belief in the importance of my journey has been a driving force behind this book, and I am indebted to your support and guidance.

To my brother, Doug, who shares in this struggle, thank you for being a source of strength and understanding. Our shared experiences have created a bond that is both unique and invaluable.

To my mother, who must wrestle with the reality of having two offspring dealing with this chronic condition, your resilience and love are truly inspiring. Thank you for your unwavering support and care.

To my niece Antoinette (Kayla) Hughes, words cannot articulate the value of your trust and support.

I extend my gratitude to all those who are dealing with and fully understand this struggle. Your courage and perseverance are a testament to the strength of the human spirit.

To all my mentors and role models, thank you for your wisdom and guidance. Your influence has shaped me into the person I am today, and I am forever grateful for your presence in my life.

Table of Contents

INTRODUCTION

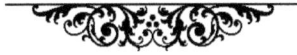

Life often takes us on an unanticipated journey, charting courses through uncharted waters that challenge our resilience and redefine our understanding of strength. This book is a testament to such a journey, my personal odyssey through the trials and triumphs of living with diabetes. More than just a chronic illness, diabetes intertwined with my life in profound ways, revealing the close relationship it shares with heart disease, particularly within the Black community.

This book delves into the depths of my experience, highlighting the intricate link between diabetes and heart disease, a connection that is especially prevalent in the Black community. As a healthcare professional, I was well-versed in the technicalities of these conditions, but facing them personally was an entirely different battle. My journey through diagnosis, acceptance, and management of diabetes transformed my life and perspective, compelling me to share my story.

This book is not only a chronicle of my struggles and victories but also a guide for those who find themselves on a similar path. It underscores the importance of recognizing early signs, seeking timely medical intervention, and understanding the broader implications of diabetes on the well-being of the heart. I hope this book brings you a sense of perspective and solace.

As you embark on this journey with me, I hope my story inspires awareness, resilience, and a proactive approach to health. Life, as I have learned, is full of unexpected twists, but it is in facing these challenges that we find our true strength.

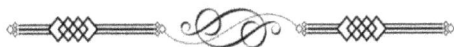

A Matter of The Heart

My Unexpected Journey with Diabetes

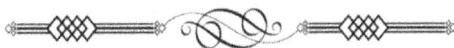

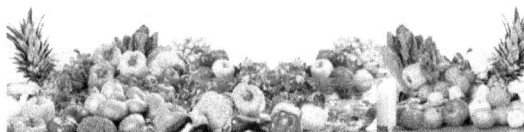

CHAPTER ONE

MY NEW BEGINNING

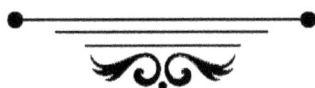

It was the summer of 1999, before the time in our history which became known as Y2K. An exciting time for me.

Why, you may ask.

I was a brand-new husband, a newlywed. I was on cloud nine, excited about my new life. My wife was expecting our first child, I was glowing in my new and invigorating circumstances. Life was indeed good. What I discovered and was about to find out is that life is like a box of chocolates, and surprises are bound to occur. As I prepared for the arrival of our child, I noticed something odd. I had always prided myself on my health, knowledge, and how I took care of myself. Yet, despite my love for food and a robust appetite, I found myself inexplicably losing weight. My clothes hung loosely, a fact that initially seemed like a benign curiosity rather than a cause for concern. I brushed off these early signs, attributing them to my active lifestyle and perhaps a faster metabolism. As time went on, I noticed my clothes getting even bigger on me. I wasn't actively trying to lose weight. I loved to eat and had a ravenous appetite. But strangely, I was not gaining any weight. But instead, I was losing weight at a significant clip. I didn't really think too much of it, as I loved biking and staying active. But I started to notice other strange occurrences. I craved sweets. Pop or Soda, which ever region you frequent, became my seductive ally. Welches Grape was my favorite. I would drink that stuff by the liters like no tomorrow.

Every day I had my fix. Days went by, turning into weeks, and I kept on drinking like a lush. So much so, I attracted the attention of my wife, who would question me frequently as to why I drank so much of it. My wife, supportive but observant, began to question my unusual drinking habits even more, prompting me to dismiss her concerns with casual explanations about having a sweet tooth like anyone else. My annoyance grew with each inquiry. I blew it off as no big deal. I just had a sweet tooth, I would say. Doesn't everybody? Again, not thinking anything was out of the ordinary, I went on with my life. Enjoying my new married life and preparing for the arrival of our child, life was good.

But the weight loss continued, and I began to get concerned. I felt fine as my appetite was strong, but I couldn't gain any weight. My new in-laws even noticed my weight loss. Especially my sister in-law. I would always make excuses as to what may be going on. I was the health professional, you know, and I always used that as collateral.

Excuses became the norm. I had sunk deeper into a state of personal denial. Who was I really fooling? You see, I was three years into my new career as a Cardiovascular Perfusionist Clinician. I was a Johns Hopkins graduate and that carried much weight, even in the smaller city of Toledo, Ohio. I spent many hours in the hospital participating in Open Heart Surgery. We had a very busy practice. We would participate in many cases of patients of all ages in need of cardiac surgical intervention. We also would assist with heart failure support; some patients needing Heart Assist devices on which we would provide 24-hour support until they were transferred to Transplant Centers for further evaluation. I worked many hours on and off calls. I was moving up in the hospital, gaining the confidence of the Surgeons, Anesthesia, nursing staff, and my peers. I was making a name for myself in my young career. It was exciting yet stressful, knowing the reality that someone's life was in my very hands. But as I was gaining experience in my new career, things began to take an unexpected twist. My life was about to dramatically change.

Having attained valuable training and experience in anatomy and physiology and learning about the human body, I was well-versed in what I was about to encounter from a technical standpoint. I knew the data well, but it was for my patients, not for me. I must provide context for what I am about to share. I was happy and content. But things began to transition in my life. I began to learn that what you read in a book can sometimes be muffled by what you experience. What am I talking about? I noticed subtle changes in my health. As I began to question what I am dealing with, my stark reality started to become my detriment. Sometimes a little knowledge can be a hindrance. I started to rationalize a lot. I sank into a deeper state of denial. I didn't want to know at first or even bother to investigate what may be going on. But the denial was no longer warranted. As a skilled perfusion clinician, I was beginning to recognize however that something was seriously wrong. These newly bizarre occurrences started to become more frequent. The thirst, less subtle but now persistent, continued. A growing thirst that seemed unquenchable, a craving for sugary drinks like Welches Grape soda that I indulged in daily without a second thought.

My wife, now started to question me even more persistently. She began to highlight further my unusual drinking habits, prompting me to dismiss her concerns with casual explanations about having a sweet tooth like anyone else. This is what piqued my curiosity and concern. I began to suffer frequent urination. I was thirsty constantly. Always drinking something, although my activity level didn't really change. How odd!! With all that going on, I still was losing weight. As I became more perplexed, so did my Inquisitiveness. I began to ask around to my colleagues at the hospital. I really didn't want to know, but my symptoms persisted. I began to recognize I could no longer play the denial game. I needed to get to the bottom of it. After an intense personal struggle, I broke down and went to the local drug store to purchase a glucose urinalysis test kit. To be honest with you, I didn't even know they existed. Never paid that much attention. I grabbed one and carefully read the instructions. It seemed easy enough. I went home and tested myself privately. I even whispered a prayer for a negative outcome. Well, the instructions were simple enough. This was a huge moment for me. Well, I was to just add my sample to the cup and see what happens. No big deal.

After adding the sample, I waited with bated breath, praying for a miracle. I must say however, some consternation and mixed feelings. I was hoping for a miracle but also wondering, if this is negative, what else could be triggering my symptoms? A lot was going through my mind. Hesitancy, yet the need for closure. Was I right after all? Enough with the back and forth, the moment of truth had finally arrived. I followed the instructions, added my sample and waited. Peering at the indicator, I watched carefully. Within minutes I realized to my chagrin, my unsuspected horror was confirmed. Dreadfully, my greatest fear was realized. Less than one year into my marriage, I suspected and now an over-the-counter drug store home test confirmed my greatest suspicion. I am now dealing with potentially juvenile-onset diabetes. My heart was broken. I knew very well the dynamic this would create. Reluctantly but prudently, I made an appointment with my healthcare practitioner to confirm.

I made the appointment quietly trying not to raise suspicion to my unsuspicious wife. What was I to do? How could I come to grips with this? How could I tell her what this would mean? After being confirmed via a blood test by my doctor, I was devastated and became very angry. I was not exactly a health nut, but I did try to take great care of myself. As a healthcare professional, I even shared knowledge on health doing numerous presentations at area churches and organizations before this occurrence. When the test confirmed my fears, my world shattered. Less than a year into my marriage, with plans for a new baby and a future full of promise, I was confronted with the reality of a chronic illness. The diagnosis of diabetes, initially suspected and then confirmed by a doctor, plunged me into a whirlwind of emotions—devastation, anger, and a profound sense of injustice. Life throws many twists, doesn't it? How could this happen to me? I questioned God many times, asking for a reprieve. Why me, Lord? Why did You let this happen? I had sunk into a mini-state of depression, trying to make sense of it all. As someone who had dedicated my professional life to healthcare, who had stood beside patients facing life-threatening surgeries and chronic conditions, I now faced the stark reality of being on the other side. I questioned why this was happening to me, pleading with a higher power for answers that seemed elusive. I didn't know how to break it to my wife. We had so much to look forward to. So much planning for our first child. We were planning trips. We were ready for the new life we chose. So much excitement and anticipation. How could this be? After much consternation and deliberation, I knew it was time to let my wife know.

After thoughtful consideration, knowing there will never be a good time, I reluctantly shared the news with her. Although I could tell the enormity of my situation was not a shocker to her, I felt a sense of relief knowing she knew, even though I knew deep down, this unfortunate condition lay dormant in her mind. We are all aware of it, but we knew very little about the trek we will share. Time will tell going forward as she will become fully aware of the challenges this condition would cause. My condition would be met with unanticipated twists. The hardest part was sharing the news with my wife, knowing that our lives would now be forever altered by this diagnosis. It was a moment of vulnerability and fear, yet in that moment, I found a strange comfort in sharing the burden. Together, we began to navigate the unknown waters of managing diabetes, a journey that would eventually evolve from Type 2 to Type 1 diabetes, requiring insulin dependence. I knew deep down my life would be forever changed. Such is the life of a newly onset diabetic.

Off we go into the turbulent uncharted waters. The beginning of a new era. To be continued . . .

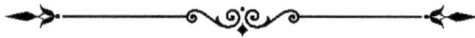

Reflection Question:

What signs or symptoms in your own life have you overlooked or downplayed, thinking they were insignificant? How did you eventually confront them?

Practical Application:

Pay attention to changes in your body and don't dismiss unusual symptoms. Regular health check-ups and proactive health screenings can help detect potential issues early, allowing for timely intervention and management.

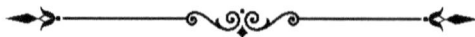

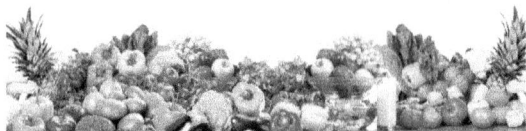

CHAPTER TWO

MY NEW UNKNOWN

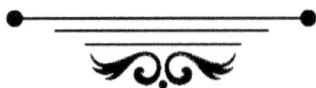

Once the dust began to settle after these new diagnoses, it was time for reflection. I never considered myself an unhealthy eater. In most of my young life, I was burdened with allergies to many different foods, so it wasn't like I was eating cupcakes and cookies continuously. I ate reasonably healthy. After my confirmation, I was advised to seek a diabetic educator and get under the care of an endocrinologist. My decisions were tempered but I knew better. I must seek to manage this to the best of my ability. As a religious man, I kept a prayer in my heart. Still wondering *why, me.* Trying not to feel too sorry for myself. But although it was a battle, mentally to fight my anger and frustration, I knew that I must press forward with my life. Pouting proved fruitless. I witnessed the birth of my first child. That gave me a reprieve. Seeing our first child was motivation to keep pressing on and fight my intense emotions. Diabetes is a full-time condition. It requires constant monitoring and management. I was aware of the myriad of complications and consequences it can cause. I made up my mind to push through my emotional stalemate and fight. I was angry for many years, but after much prayer, I realized I must get past this by God's grace. He allowed it, so there must be a purpose in all of this.

I loved my wife dearly and cannot blame her or anyone for my affliction. Despite my grief, I knew I had to shake out of it. Regardless of this diagnosis, I was still a husband and father, and I wanted to be healthy and be there for my other children and my wife. Life can throw you many setbacks and challenges. But I have discovered that in this life, crap happens. I cannot stop living because of a setback. What example is that to my wife and my children? I decided to gather as much info on this condition as I could. I listed questions for my diabetic educator. I investigated what foods to eat. What foods did I need to avoid? I'm not going to say this was easy. That would be a lie. But I must say it was necessary. Life matters: change your perspective. I measured where I was and needed to be, and decided, by God's grace, I will keep pressing on. I had too much living to forgo. Yes, I am an insulin dependent Type 1 diabetic. But I am alive. With good management and control, I can beat this. I can pursue dreams. I can grow as a husband and father. I'm still around to smell the roses that are plentiful. I had to get past the hurt and just live. I prayed and felt a sense of calm and purpose.

As I thought, I am not the only case of diabetes in this world. Use this condition to grow and even inspire other diabetics that are not familiar with this condition as I am. I needed to refocus on the positives. I am not dead yet. Life is for the living. God will be my strength. I really can't do this alone. This is why I wanted to share my testimony. I am not the only one dealing with this condition. In fact, I'm more than surprised to find out how many are dealing with it. With worsening symptoms as I have manifested. Yes, I reflected on where I could have been. Yes, I am a diabetic, but I am alive and able to function and fulfill my calling. I settled into a routine. Blood sugar checks, making sure I get regular checkups. My family needs a father, I need my family. It's now on me. I pledged not to be defeated by this dreadful condition. Prayer and perseverance are needed. I bathed myself in prayer and marched forward. This level of detail was new for me. It took time getting used to the regimen. I had to estimate my caloric intake. I had to measure out my insulin dose. Timing was important to make sure my glucose readings didn't get too high. This was truly a moment. Wow, I knew it would be difficult, but man!!! This was intense. I had to watch what I ate; it was very complex carbohydrates, starchy, which took longer to break down. Measuring out fruits versus vegetables. I was already a vegetarian so how does that get mixed into the equation? I couldn't eat late like I used to sometimes. You know, the late Saturday night snacks. As things settled in, I thought I was on top of it. But one night, all that changed. I received a call from my mother that my dad was heading to the hospital. He has had some health challenges but was in otherwise good health. He was taken to the Emergency Room at the University of Michigan Hospital. I felt the need to drive up and check on him. We were living in Ohio at the time. I went to head up north but mysteriously couldn't find my keys. I must have dropped them on the floor of the car. As I pondered their whereabouts, and in my present condition, my wife peeked into the garage and inquired as to what was going on. I must have been out there for a minute. I'm not sure if I even answered her but she knew I wanted to drive up to see my dad. I must have looked distraught over my father's condition. So, she decided to drive me up there. As we got on the expressway, I started to get confused. I expressed to her that something was off. So, instead of going up to Michigan, we were going to go to the nearest hospital for me.

At this point, I was confused and could provide no assistance for getting there. My wife was not familiar with that part of town, and I had the GPS. Still unaware of my actions, I tried to give directions but passed out multiple times. We got off trying to get assistance and finally ended up at a station off the beaten path. I was totally out of it at this time. My wife can fill in the rest of this story. When I came too, I was in the back of an ambulance and told what I just endured. As they explained to me what had happened, I was in total shock. I had undergone a diabetic hypoglycemic episode.

What did that mean you ask? My blood sugar dropped critically which caused my current situation. I was in total disbelief. I knew I was not feeling myself, but to have sugar drop to that level where I needed paramedic intervention was shocking to me. This had never happened before. I was taken to the local hospital, but once I was assessed, I was fine, and then we went home.

This was the first time something like this had ever happened to me. This whole situation was so surreal. I was aware but not aware. When your sugar drops, the best way to describe it is that you are in a dream state. You think you are aware, but you aren't. It is truly a crazy surrealistic experience. You could only relate if you ever experienced it. You can't talk. You can't reason. You can't think. You just exist, and without help, even worse can happen. This was indeed a wake-up call on many fronts. The best way to describe diabetes is for six days, you can be on your game.

But all it takes is one moment, and disaster can strike. One thing I gathered from this crazy experience is that indeed there is a God. This was not some lucky set of circumstances, but truly a Divine encounter. I would not be writing this book. God preserved my life that dreadful night. Hence, I wanted to share this testimony. I want to let people know that God is real, and He will intervene when you are totally incapable. Also, diabetes requires diligence and patience. I almost lost my life that night. But I am here to tell you my story. I am here and proud to share my experience and let others know we can do this through Him that gives us strength.

Because of the many challenges this condition can cause, I am here to shout from the mountaintop about the need to heighten awareness of diabetes. This condition has its definite pitfalls, but we can persevere and get through it. I am a witness, and we need to be made more aware of the risks, pitfalls, and ways to prevent them if possible. I came to realize this is a walk of sheer resiliency. What do I mean by that, you may ask?

According to the dictionary, resilience is an ability to recover from or adjust easily to misfortune or change. I almost lost my life, but as I stated earlier, I am here writing this book. I was never a quitter. I always fought through any adversity that came my way. You will experience this sometimes with Diabetes. There are ebbs and flows as they say. But, when you have much to live for, you press on. I pressed on. I serve a God who delivered me from my dire circumstances. Although I did not know what lied ahead in this turbulent walk, I did know and believed that God was with me every step of the way. That changed my perspective. I can now step forward in these uncharted waters with a calm assurance, I can do this. The good book says in Philippians 4:13, I can do all things through Christ who strengthens me. Well, I definitely needed strength. This is my advice to all that deal with Diabetes. You must keep pressing on the forward path. Despite the setbacks. I was always told that a setback is a setup for a comeback. I genuinely believe that. You must believe that. We march on.

In the next chapter, I will explore more, get into the need to sound the alarm, and discuss the risks involved. If we can prevent it, let's do everything in our power to do that. This is a national threat; do we have any way to reduce our risk? Let's explore the next chapter. We need to sound the alarm nationally, particularly in the Black and Brown communities. All communities are at risk, but some demographics are definite at a higher risk. Looking back, I realize how easy it is to overlook or downplay symptoms, especially when they seem insignificant or when we believe ourselves invulnerable. My journey with diabetes taught me the importance of listening to my body and not dismissing subtle changes as inconsequential.

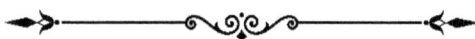

Reflection Question:

Has a significant health diagnosis or challenge ever impacted your perspective on life and your priorities? If yes, how?

Practical Application:

Take time to reflect on your own health habits and lifestyle choices. Consider seeking advice from healthcare professionals even if you feel healthy, as prevention and early detection can make a significant difference in managing health conditions effectively.

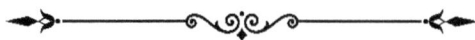

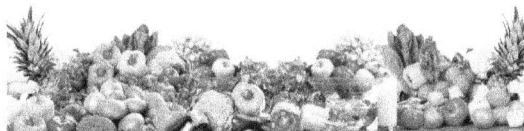

CHAPTER THREE

SOUND THE ALARM: MANAGING DIABETES IN AMERICA

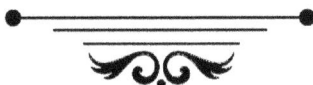

As a former Cardiovascular Perfusionist with a decade of experience in the medical field, and now a seasoned Medical Affairs professional, I've witnessed firsthand the profound impact of diabetes on individuals and our healthcare system. Diabetes isn't just a diagnosis; it's a growing epidemic that demands our attention and action. The numbers continue to grow. When I was diagnosed, I knew it would be a trek, but I had no idea how rocky it was. I have seen family and friends stricken. It hurts my heart; no pun was intended to see the level of cases manifested.

When I went to my first few visits at the Endocrinologist, it was so heartbreaking seeing the condition of many of the patients coming into the clinic. Yes, I was angry, but the reality hit me hard that we must try to beat this thing. This scourge is growing by the day. I began to wonder what I could do to get the word out and share my concerns. Being Type 1 insulin, dependent is laborious and taxing. However, when it comes to life and death, I choose life, and I'm willing to do whatever I can to improve my situation. I'm watching my kids grow up and want to see them to the finish line.

The Diabetes Epidemic: A Call to Action

The challenge is that Diabetes affects millions of Americans, with numbers rising alarmingly each year. From my vantage point in healthcare and industry, I've seen how this chronic condition not only challenges individuals but also strains our healthcare resources. Globally, diabetes has increased due to Westernization and industrialization. Diabetes is rare in traditional societies in Africa and Asia where diets are high in complex carbohydrates and starches.

The prevalence of diabetes in the United States has reached unprecedented levels, affecting people of all ages, backgrounds, and lifestyles. This is not a Black or White issue. All are at risk. According to the Centers for Disease Control, 38.4 million people of all ages—or 11.6% of the U.S. population—had diabetes. 38.1 million adults aged 18 years or older—or 14.7% of all U.S. adults—had diabetes. (See Reference Tables)

Table 1a. Estimated crude prevalence of diagnosed diabetes, undiagnosed diabetes, and total diabetes among adults aged 18 years or older, United States, 2017–2020.

Characteristic	Diagnosed diabetes Percentage (95% CI)	Undiagnosed diabetes Percentage (95% CI)	Total diabetes Percentage (95% CI)
Total	11.3 (10.3–12.5)	3.4 (2.7–4.2)	14.7 (13.2–16.4)
Age in years			
18–44	3.0 (2.4–3.7)	1.9 (1.3–2.7)	4.8 (4.0–5.9)
45–64	14.5 (12.2–17.0)	4.5 (3.3–6.0)	18.9 (16.1–22.1)
≥65	24.4 (22.1–27.0)	4.7 (3.0–7.4)	29.2 (26.4–32.1)
Sex			
Men	12.6 (11.1–14.3)	2.8 (2.0–3.9)	15.4 (13.5–17.5)
Women	10.2 (8.8–11.7)	3.9 (2.7–5.5)	14.1 (11.8–16.7)
Race-Ethnicity			
White, non-Hispanic	11.0 (9.4–12.8)	2.7 (1.7–4.2)	13.6 (11.4–16.2)
Black, non-Hispanic	12.7 (10.7–15.0)	4.7 (3.3–6.5)	17.4 (15.2–19.8)
Asian, non-Hispanic	11.3 (9.7–13.1)	5.4 (3.5–8.3)	16.7 (14.0–19.8)
Hispanic	11.1 (9.5–13.0)	4.4 (3.3–5.8)	15.5 (13.8–17.3)

Notes: CI = confidence interval. Time period 2017–2020 covers January 2017 through March 2020 only. Diagnosed diabetes was based on self-report. Undiagnosed diabetes was based on fasting plasma glucose and A1C levels among people self-reporting no diabetes. Numbers for subgroups may not add up to the total because of rounding. Age-adjusted estimates are presented in Appendix Table 1. Data source: 2017–March 2020 National Health and Nutrition Examination Survey.

Table 1b. Estimated number of adults aged 18 years or older with diagnosed diabetes, undiagnosed diabetes, and total diabetes, United States, 2021

Characteristic	Diagnosed diabetes Number in Millions (95% CI)	Undiagnosed Diabetes Number in Millions (95% CI)	Total diabetes Number in Millions (95% CI)
Total	**29.4 (26.7–32.0)**	**8.7 (7.0–10.5)**	**38.1 (34.2–42.0)**
Age in years			
18–44	3.5 (2.8–4.2)	2.2 (1.5–3.0)	5.8 (4.7–6.8)
45–64	12.0 (10.1–13.9)	3.8 (2.7–4.8)	15.8 (13.4–18.2)
≥65	13.8 (12.5–15.1)	2.7 (1.6–3.8)	16.5 (15.0–18.1)
Sex			
Men	16.1 (14.1–18.0)	3.7 (2.6–4.8)	19.8 (17.4–22.1)

Characteristic	Diagnosed diabetes Number in Millions (95% CI)	Undiagnosed Diabetes Number in Millions (95% CI)	Total diabetes Number in Millions (95% CI)
Women	13.3 (11.5–15.1)	5.0 (3.3–6.7)	18.3 (15.3–21.3)
Race-Ethnicity			
White, non-Hispanic	17.8 (15.2–20.4)	4.3 (2.4–6.1)	22.1 (18.5–25.7)
Black, non-Hispanic	4.0 (3.3–4.6)	1.4 (1.0–1.9)	5.4 (4.7–6.1)
Asian, non-Hispanic	1.8 (1.5–2.1)	0.9 (0.5–1.2)	2.7 (2.2–3.1)
Hispanic	5.0 (4.3–5.7)	1.9 (1.4–2.4)	6.9 (6.2–7.6)

Notes: CI = confidence interval. Estimated numbers for 2021 were derived from percentages for 2017–March 2020 applied to July 1, 2021, U.S. resident population estimates from the U.S. Census Bureau (See detailed methods and data sources). Diagnosed diabetes was based on self-report. Undiagnosed diabetes was based on fasting plasma glucose and A1C levels among people self-reporting no diabetes. Numbers for subgroups may not add up to the total because of rounding.

Data sources: 2017–March 2020 National Health and Nutrition Examination Survey; 2021 U.S. Census Bureau data.

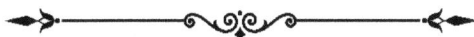

But unfortunately, we are more impacted. For both men and women, the prevalence of diagnosed diabetes was highest among American Indian and Alaska Native adults (13.6%), followed by non-Hispanic Black adults (12.1%). In 2019, non-Hispanic blacks were twice as likely as non-Hispanic whites to die from diabetes. In 2018, African American adults were 60 percent more likely than non-Hispanic white adults to be diagnosed with diabetes by a physician. Also, in 2019, non-Hispanic blacks were 2.5 times more likely to be hospitalized with diabetes and associated long-term complications than non-Hispanic whites. In 2019, non-Hispanic blacks were 3.2 times more likely to be diagnosed with end-stage renal disease as compared to non-Hispanic whites. This is a big deal that needs to be addressed.

When I'm sitting in the clinics, we many times are missing or in low attendance. This is because racial and ethnic disparities in health and health care remain a persistent challenge in the United States. Unfortunately, as reported by the Kaiser Family Foundation, the COVID-19 pandemic's uneven impact on people of color drew increased attention to inequities in health and health care, which have been documented for decades and reflect longstanding structural and systemic inequities rooted in historical and ongoing racism and discrimination. That bothers me very much. We have a higher incidence of this chronic condition, with less access to healthcare. I realize that far too often for us, a trip to the doctor is a trip to urgent care or the ED. We are not being followed like we should. That will lead to major complications in the long run and even poorer outcomes. Mortality rates soar as we let this slip past us in the prime time of our lives.

According to a Pew Research Center Study, Minorities point to the health care system as contributing to the problem, noting that 49% cite a major reason why minorities generally have worse health outcomes is because health care providers are less likely to give our lower socioeconomic population the most advanced medical care. A roughly equal share (47%) says hospitals and medical centers are giving lower priority to their well-being, and also a major reason for differing health outcomes. This unfortunately, further exacerbates an already taxing problem. Diabetes is a chronic condition with potentially serious complications, but this is not a death sentence, and we must be vigilant on all accounts.

Managing Diabetes: A User-Friendly Approach

Managing diabetes starts with understanding. Whether you're newly diagnosed or have been living with diabetes for years, education and awareness are key. In my role as a Medical Affairs professional, I've had the privilege of helping to bridge the gap between medical innovation and patient care. This book aims to provide a user-friendly guide to understanding diabetes for all demographics, offering practical tips and insights that empower individuals to take control of their health. I have the privilege to work for a company that develops therapeutics for peripheral vascular disease. A very common byproduct of diabetes. I will explain this more in the next chapter but there are ways to reduce our risk for extreme complications.

First, what is Diabetes?

Well, sugar (glucose) is the basic energy source or fuel for the cells of the body. Glucose provides the energy to move, think, etc. Insulin is a hormone, produced by the pancreas that has the password or the key to open the door of your cells to let glucose in. Diabetes occurs when blood glucose levels rise because:

1. for some reason, the body is not making (enough) insulin.
2. insulin gets to the door of the cell, but the cell resists, and the door does not open.

As a consequence, when glucose has trouble getting into your cells, you have no energy and feel tired.

When glucose can't enter your cells, it builds up in your bloodstream. As glucose gets concentrated in the blood, it passes through the kidneys and enters the urine. As it passes through your kidneys, glucose takes all the water it can get, thus frequent urination and thirst. As the cells begin to starve for energy, you can lose weight as I experienced in my early onset. These are the classic symptoms to look for.

Bridging the Gap: From Perfusionist to Patient

My background as a Cardiovascular Perfusionist has uniquely positioned me to understand the intricacies of health management. From monitoring patients during cardiac surgeries to advocating for better patient outcomes in the industry, I've seen how proactive healthcare can make a difference. The United States has the highest health expenditures of any developed country worldwide; however, only about 8% of Americans currently undergo routine preventive screenings.

As a result, the US loses about $55 billion US dollars (USD) each year due to missed prevention opportunities. The earlier you identify a problem, the better the outcomes. Now, as someone living with diabetes, I bring a dual perspective to the table — as a healthcare professional and as a patient navigating the challenges of a chronic condition. Yes, I was angry, but now I'm extremely motivated. I must let you all know that we cannot allow this condition to rule us. We must fight for our lives. We must do all we can to survive. As the saying goes, prevention is worth a pound of cure. I will highlight later in this book ways to minimize, reduce, or prevent this dreadful but doable condition. I will discuss later in this book eight key health principles that will aid in this struggle.

A Message of Hope and Empowerment

Living with diabetes is a journey, not a destination. It requires diligence, education, and support from healthcare providers, loved ones, and the broader community. Through this book, I hope to inspire and encourage others facing similar challenges. Diabetes is manageable, and with the right tools and mindset, it is possible to live a full and healthy life.

Taking Charge of Your Health

The growing incidence of diabetes in the United States is a clarion call for action. As someone who has dedicated his career to healthcare, I urge you to take charge of your health. Whether you're a healthcare professional, a patient, or a concerned family member, together we can make a difference in the fight against diabetes. Let's turn awareness into action and empower individuals to live their best lives despite diabetes. But we must now focus on our most vulnerable populations.

As we jump into chapter 4, I will explore diabetes's impact on the United State community and its minority populations.

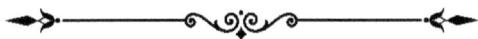

Reflection Question:

What steps can you take today to increase your awareness of diabetes and its potential impact on your life or the lives of loved ones?

Practical Application:

As 1 in 3 American adults have prediabetes. Consider scheduling a health check-up to assess your risk factors for diabetes, such as blood sugar levels, blood pressure, and weight. Educate yourself about healthy lifestyle choices that can help prevent or manage diabetes effectively. You can take an online survey or test to determine your risk. This test assesses your risk by age, family history, blood pressure, race/ethnicity, wellness, gender and BMI. Early detection is key.

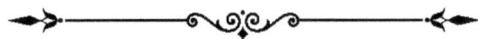

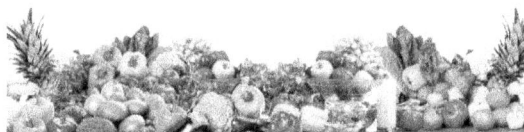

CHAPTER FOUR

DIABETES AND CARDIOVASCULAR DISEASE IN THE BLACK COMMUNITY

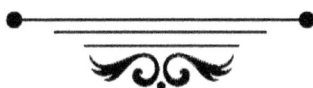

For those who are religious, the Bible states that people will perish for a lack of knowledge. Unfortunately, this has shown itself with amazing accuracy. I have witnessed firsthand the alarming intersection of diabetes and cardiovascular disease, particularly within our American or US community. In this chapter, we will explore the profound impact of diabetes on heart health, the shared risk factors, and strategies for prevention and management.

The Alarming Statistics

Diabetes has emerged as a significant health challenge, especially among Minorities. The American Heart Association considers diabetes one of the major controllable risk factors for cardiovascular disease (CVD) for all demographics. In fact, people living with Type 2 diabetes are more likely to develop and die from cardiovascular diseases, such as heart attacks, strokes, and heart failure, than people who don't have diabetes. The link, according to the National Institute of Diabetes and Digestive and Kidney Diseases (NIDDK), is high blood glucose from diabetes can damage your blood vessels and the nerves that control your heart and blood vessels. Over time, this damage can lead to heart disease.

People with diabetes tend to develop heart disease at a younger age than people without diabetes. Adults with diabetes are nearly twice as likely to have heart disease or stroke as adults without diabetes. According to recent studies, approximately 33% of African Americans diagnosed with diabetes also suffer from heart disease. The pattern holds similarly for other groups: White Americans with diabetes: Cardiovascular Disease (CVD) appears in ~4.2%, roughly 46% of diabetics. For Hispanics: CVD in 3.8%, about 25% of those with diabetes. Asian Americans: CVD in 2.8%, representing roughly 24% of diabetics. It is interesting to note, Type 2 diabetes affects minority communities more than other groups. A potential connection is differences in health status, access to health care, and income which are largely the main drivers of these health disparities. Social and economic barriers make accessible health care more difficult for many underprivileged people. High healthcare costs coupled with lower insurance rates mean that many minorities cannot afford quality medical care and prescription medications, so conditions such as diabetes are not managed as well as they could be and subsequently result in poorer outcomes. This staggering statistic underscores the critical need for heightened awareness and initiative-taking management of these interconnected conditions. Why are we so susceptible? Many theories are at play.

Leading Cause of Mortality

In both men and women of color diagnosed with diabetes, heart disease stands out as the leading cause of death, often manifesting as heart attacks or strokes. The mortality rates among diabetic individuals due to heart disease are notably higher compared to those without diabetes. This stark reality necessitates a multifaceted approach to address both the prevention and treatment of diabetes and cardiovascular conditions.

Shared Risk Factors

One of the most striking parallels between diabetes and heart disease lies in their shared risk factors. Obesity, characterized by excess body weight, particularly around the abdomen, is a significant contributor to both conditions. High blood pressure (hypertension) further exacerbates the risk, leading to complications such as coronary artery disease and stroke.

The Role of Lifestyle Modifications

In combating the dual epidemics of diabetes and cardiovascular disease, lifestyle modifications play a pivotal role. Adopting a healthy diet rich in fruits, vegetables, whole grains, and lean proteins can help manage blood sugar levels and reduce the risk of heart disease. Regular physical activity not only aids in weight management but also enhances cardiovascular fitness and overall well-being.

Empowering the Community:

Education and awareness are vital in empowering individuals, families, and communities to take proactive steps towards better health outcomes. Initiatives that promote regular health screenings, diabetes management programs, and culturally sensitive interventions are essential in bridging the gap and reducing disparities in healthcare access and outcomes.

Looking Ahead

As we navigate the complex landscape of diabetes and

cardiovascular disease, ongoing research and advancements in medical technology offer hope for improved prevention, early detection, and treatment options. By fostering collaboration between healthcare providers, policymakers, and community leaders, we can strive towards a future where all individuals, regardless of race or background, can live healthier lives.

The convergence of diabetes and cardiovascular disease presents a formidable challenge, particularly within the lower socioeconomic and minority communities. By addressing shared risk factors, promoting healthy lifestyles, and enhancing community engagement, we can work towards reducing the burden of these diseases and fostering a healthier future for generations to come.

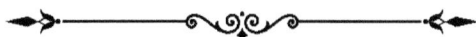

Reflection Question:

How can communities and healthcare providers collaborate to better educate, and to support minority populations affected by diabetes and cardiovascular disease?

Practical Application:

Get involved in community health initiatives or support groups focused on diabetes awareness and prevention, particularly those targeting minority communities. Advocate for culturally sensitive healthcare programs and resources that address the specific needs of diverse populations. Here are a few examples of groups that you may partner with. They have awareness campaigns you can participate in.

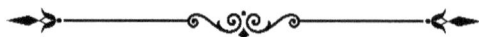

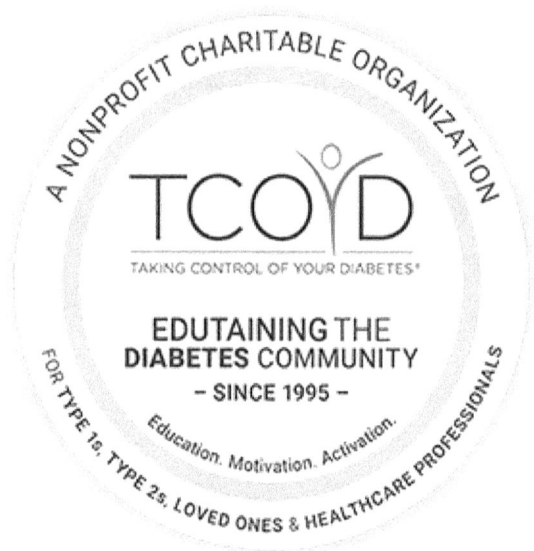

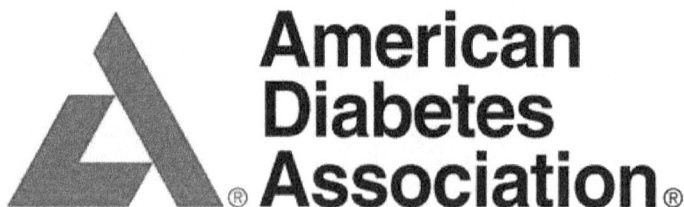

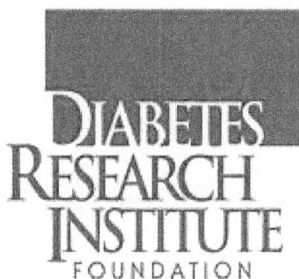

The Best Hope for a Cure®

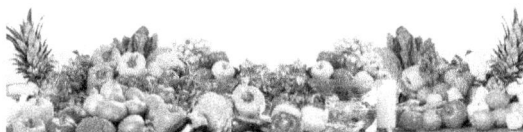

CHAPTER FIVE

A JOURNEY OF RESILIENCE AND HOPE

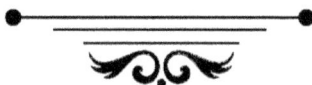

As I reflect on my journey battling diabetes, I am reminded of the profound impact it has had not only on my life but on countless others, especially within the Black community where the burden of diabetes and heart disease looms large. I've witnessed firsthand the devastating effects of these diseases. Yet, amidst the challenges, I've also discovered a path forward, a set of principles that have guided me and can empower others to reclaim their health and vitality.

We are in a battle for our wellness, and we must try to change our trajectory. The eight key health principles I propose are fresh air, water, sunshine, rest, exercise, a healthy diet, temperance, and trust in God. They are not merely suggestions but pillars of transformation. Fresh air reminds us to embrace nature's healing power, while water nourishes and purifies our bodies from within. Sunshine, often overlooked, offers essential vitamin D and lifts our spirits. Rest allows our bodies to rejuvenate, which is essential for managing stress and maintaining optimal health.

Exercise, in its myriad forms, strengthens our hearts and bodies, promoting longevity and vitality. A brisk walk well does you well. Coupled with a healthy diet rich in whole foods and balanced nutrients, it forms the foundation of disease prevention and management. Practicing temperance in all aspects of life—moderation in habits, balanced emotions, and disciplined choices—fosters harmony within ourselves and our communities. Above all, trust in God anchors us in faith and resilience, providing strength through adversity and guiding us toward holistic wellness. These principles, woven into the fabric of everyday life, offer a roadmap to combatting diabetes and heart disease, not as isolated individuals but as a united community striving for health equity and empowerment.

HERE ARE PRACTICAL BENEFITS TO THE FOLLOWING: THE 8 HEALTH PRINCIPLES.

1. **Fresh Air**:
   - Helps improve oxygen intake, supports respiratory health, and boosts overall well-being by providing a clean environment.
   - 25 minutes: Go out for a stroll and take some deep breaths. You could even eat your lunch outside or take a phone call or meeting outdoors.
   - When we're in urban environments or the office all day, we can experience sensory overload, resulting in tension and mental fatigue. Studies have shown that our minds and bodies relax in a natural setting. This increases feelings of pleasure and can help us concentrate and focus more effectively, according to studies in the National Library of Medicine.

2. **Water**:
   - Essential for hydration, helps in digestion, nutrient absorption, circulation, and regulates body temperature.
   - How much water should you drink a day? Most people need about four to six cups of plain water each

day. But it may be surprising to learn that water intake is an individualized number.

- While the daily four-to-six cup rule is for generally healthy people, that amount differs based on how much water they take in from other beverages and food sources. Also, certain health conditions, medications, activity levels, and ambient temperature influence total daily water intake.

- Unfortunately, many of us aren't getting enough to drink, especially older adults. We'll help you understand how much water you need to drink in a day to stay healthy.

3. Sunshine:

- Promotes vitamin D synthesis, which is crucial for bone health, supports mood regulation, and enhances immune function.

- 5 minutes: Stand outside with the sun on your face or take off your shoes to feel the grass in between your toes. If the weather isn't great, take a few minutes to gaze out a window at the scenery outside.

- How much is needed? In general, scientists think 5 to 15 minutes -- up to 30 if you're dark-skinned -- is about right to get the most out of it without causing any health problems. You can stay out longer and get the same effect if you use sunscreen. Talk to your doctor about what's right for you.

4. **Rest**:

○ Allows for physical and mental recovery, promotes better cognitive function, and supports overall stress management.

○ Most adults need 7 or more hours of sleep each night. It's also important to get good-quality sleep on a regular schedule so you feel rested when you wake up.

○ Kids need even more sleep than adults:

○ Teens (age 13 to 17 years) need to sleep between 8 and 10 hours each night.

○ School-aged children (age 6 to 12 years) need to sleep between 9 and 12 hours each night.

○ Preschoolers (age 3 to 5 years) need to sleep between 10 and 13 hours a day, including naps.

○ Toddlers (age 1 to 2 years) need to sleep between 11 and 14 hours a day, including naps.

○ Babies (age 4 to 12 months) need to sleep between 12

and 16 hours a day, including naps.

o Newborns (age 0 to 3 months) need to sleep between 14 and 17 hours a day.

5. **Exercise**:

o Improves cardiovascular health, strengthens muscles and bones, enhances flexibility and coordination, and supports mental well-being.

o The CDC recently report three key benefits of exercise and being active. Physical activity has many immediate and long-term benefits.

o Physical activity helps you immediately feel better, function better, and sleep better.

o Adults who sit less and do any amount of moderate-to vigorous-intensity physical activity gain some health benefits.

o It can reduce your risk of major illnesses, such as coronary heart disease, stroke, type 2 diabetes, and cancer, and lower your risk of early death by up to 30%.

6. **Healthy Diet**:

o Provides essential nutrients, vitamins, and minerals

necessary for bodily functions, supports optimal weight management, and reduces the risk of chronic diseases.

o   Dr. Neal Barnard, MD, FACC, who is an Adjunct Professor of Medicine at the George Washington University School of Medicine in Washington, DC, and President of the Physicians Committee for Responsible Medicine. has developed a revolutionary approach to addressing Diabetes. He noted that a diet consisting of High complex carbohydrates, high plant fiber diet (HCF), and a low-fat diet, 70% of calories from complex carbohydrates, 21% from protein, and 9% from fat plant fiber from whole grain cereals and breads (40%); starchy vegetables, such as beans, corn or peas (20%), other vegetables (31%); fruits (9%) dramatically reduced insulin resistance and improved overall health. Conventional diabetes diets do not lead to reduced insulin use. But Diets with 70 to 85% complex carbohydrates, and 10% or less fat produce improved glucose metabolism. When diabetics resume traditional eating after 2 or 3 weeks on an HCF diet, their need for insulin returns. Diet is key in the control, management, or even reversal of diabetes.

7. **Temperance**:

   o Encourages moderation and self-control in all aspects of life, promoting balance and preventing excesses that can lead to health issues.

   o Temperance is a state of mind wherein you seek to practice balance with your body and your passions. As stated by Dr. Randy Bivens, a Loma Linda Graduate and President of the Life and Health Network, "The true key to living a temperate lifestyle lies in our minds. We need to learn to safeguard our thoughts and carefully monitor our emotions. If you're the type to give rise to anger easily, take a few deep breaths and learn the power of forgiveness. If you're prone to bragging, give way to more humble conversation. If you're the judgmental type, give compassion or empathy a try. Think of your mind as a springboard for all of your actions. If you can learn to use your mind carefully and wisely, you will have won the battle against intemperance."

8. **Trust in God**:

   o Provides emotional and spiritual support, encourages positive coping mechanisms, and promotes a sense of purpose and inner peace, which can contribute to overall health and well-being. The Bible has provided our first template on how to live and even what to eat. Good health practices begin by adhering and studying its biblical principles.

o Together, these principles form a holistic approach to health that focuses on both physical and spiritual well-being. In sharing my story, I hope to inspire others to embrace these principles, to take charge of their health journeys, and to advocate for systemic changes that promote wellness for all. Together, we can stem the tide of diabetes and heart disease, fostering a future where health disparities diminish and hope flourish.

Certainly! Here's a closing chapter that encapsulates the journey of resilience and hope in the face of diabetes. As I reflect on the winding path that diabetes has carved through my life, I am struck by the resilience that has grown within me. It has been a journey of challenges, victories, and profound lessons that have shaped not just my health but my entire perspective on life.

Living with diabetes taught me resilience in its purest form. It demanded discipline, consistency, and unwavering commitment to self-care. There were days when the weight of managing this condition felt overwhelming, yet each hurdle became a stepping-stone towards greater understanding and strength. Through the highs and lows, I discovered the profound power of hope. It was hope that pushed me forward on days when my body felt weary and my spirit faltered. Hope became my companion, whispering that with each new day came a chance to better manage my health, to inspire others facing similar battles, and to contribute to the ongoing journey of medical knowledge and patient advocacy. This journey wasn't mine alone. Alongside me stood a support network of loved ones, healthcare professionals, and fellow warriors in the fight against diabetes. Their encouragement, guidance, and shared experiences illuminated the path forward and reaffirmed that I was never alone in this battle.

As I continue my journey in this chapter of my life, I do so with gratitude for the resilience that diabetes cultivated within me and the hope that continues to light my way. It is a journey that has taught me invaluable lessons about the power of perseverance, the importance of self-care, and the beauty of embracing life's challenges with courage and optimism. May my experiences serve as a beacon of hope for others navigating similar paths. Let us continue to forge ahead with resilience, guided by the unwavering belief that through strength and hope, we can overcome any obstacle that comes our way.

Nevertheless, be reminded that our journey towards health is ongoing, marked by resilience, compassion, and a commitment to ourselves and each other. Let us walk this path together, guided by these principles, towards a healthier, brighter future.

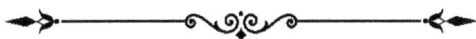

***

Reflection Question:

How has your perception of resilience evolved through the challenges you've faced, and how can you apply this understanding to managing your health journey?

Practical Application:

Take time to reflect on moments in your life where resilience played a significant role in overcoming obstacles. Identify specific strategies or coping mechanisms like:

1) Noticing when you feel stressed,
2) Taking time to relax,
3) Getting active and eating healthy,
4) Finding solutions to problems you're having,
5) Talking to friends and family,

that helps you navigate difficult times. Consider how you can integrate these lessons into your approach to managing diabetes or any other health challenges you may face. Join diabetes focus groups online like on Facebook. There are many blogs and chatrooms that discuss diabetes treatment and shared experiences. It helps you to realize you are not walking alone.

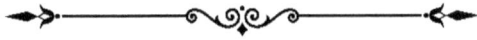

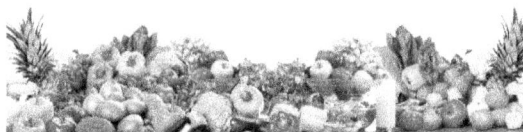

CHAPTER SIX

REDUCING RISK AND MANAGING DIABETES EFFECTIVELY

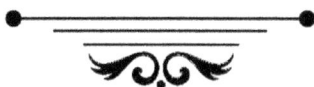

In this final chapter of my journey battling diabetes, I want to delve deeper into practical strategies for reducing the risk of diabetes and effectively managing the condition. Diabetes is a formidable opponent, but armed with knowledge and proactive measures, we can significantly impact our health outcomes and quality of life.

REDUCING RISK FACTORS

Prevention is key when it comes to diabetes. While some risk factors like genetics are beyond our control, many lifestyle factors play a crucial role in either increasing or decreasing our risk. Risk reduction encompasses many of the strategies listed in earlier chapters needed to reduce risk and stay ahead of this condition. Here are proactive steps you can take to reduce your risk of developing diabetes:

a. Maintain Healthy Weight: Obesity is a significant risk factor for diabetes. Adopting a balanced diet and incorporating regular physical activity can help achieve and maintain a healthy weight.

b. Dietary intake of extra fat in the cell paves the way for diabetes in the future. Even if slim, it is possible to have extra fat building up in muscle cells. Fat can start accumulating in the cells years before diabetes shows up. When we reduce our intake of fat, fat inside the cell dissipates, and normal cell function returns.

c. Research reveals that eating a diet low in fat can reduce the buildup of fat within the cell.

d. By changing our diet, we can dramatically reduce our chances of getting diabetes and its complications.

Eat a Balanced Diet: Focus on whole foods such as fruits, vegetables, whole grains, lean proteins, and healthy fats. Limit processed foods, sugary beverages, and excessive intake of refined carbohydrates.

Whole food diets consisting of whole grains, vegetables, legumes, and fruit, no animal products, no added oils, and no sugar or refined carbohydrates (such as white bread or refined pasta) are excellent choices to minimize health risks, especially diabetes. (See the following tables.)

The New 4 Food Group

Whole Grains

Whole grain pasta, brown rice, bran cereal, whole grain bread: 8 servings/day

A serving: ½ cup cooked grain; 1 oz. dry cereal; 1 slice bread

Legumes

Beans, peas, fat free soy products: 3 servings/day

A serving: ½ cup cooked beans; 4 oz. tofu; 8 oz soy milk

Vegetables

Sweet potatoes, broccoli, cauliflower, spinach, squash etc,: 4+ servings/day

A serving: 1 cup raw or ½ cup cooked vegetables

Fruits

Bananas, pears, mangoes, oranges, etc.: 3+ servings/dy

A serving: 1 piece raw fruit, ½ cup chopped fruit; ½ cup cooked fruit or juice

Barnard, *Reversing Diabetes*, 2007

What is 9 servings a day?

Morning

Counts as
1
3/4 cup

Counts as
1
medium-size

Mid-Day

Counts as
2
2 cups

Counts as
1
medium-size

Evening

Counts as
2
1 cup

Counts as
1
1/2

Counts as
1
1/2 cup

Cancer Institute

ChooseMyPlate.gov

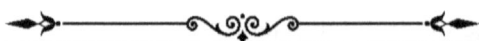

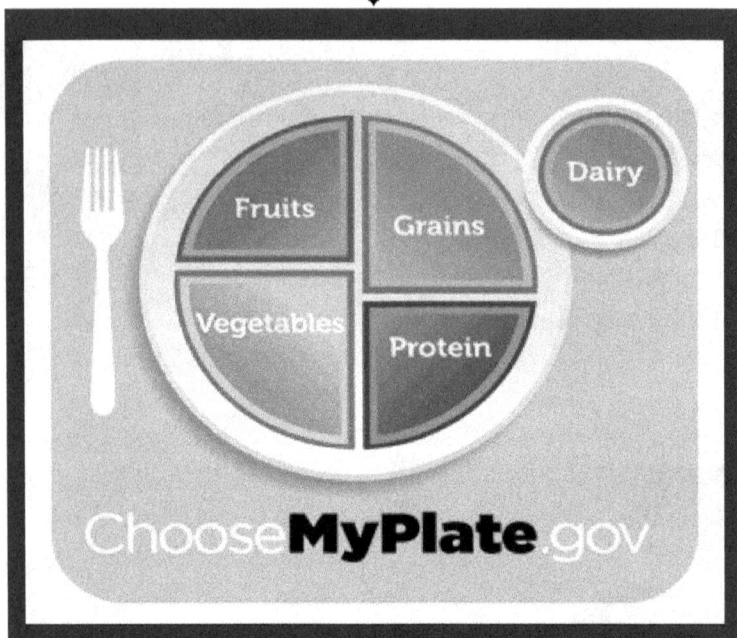

Take Home Lessons

- About one-third of people with diabetes are unaware that they have the disease
- Focus on key principles:
  - -- more whole grain
  - -- more food as grown
  - -- more fruits and vegetables
  - -- drastic reduction of all fat

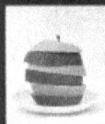

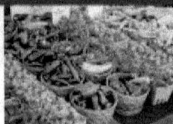

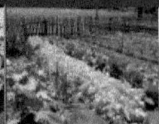

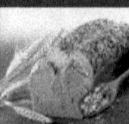

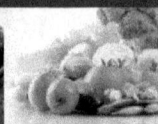

- Focus on making changes for the long term

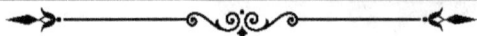

e. Exercise Regularly: Physical activity not only helps with weight management but also improves insulin sensitivity. Aim for at least 150 minutes of moderate-intensity exercise per week.

f. Regular physical activity can help you maintain a healthy weight by increasing the number of calories your body uses for energy. This can help you create a calorie deficit when combined with reducing your calorie intake, which can result in weight loss. The amount of physical activity you need to maintain a healthy weight varies by person, but adults should try to get at least:

g. 150 minutes per week: Of moderate-intensity aerobic activity, such as walking, running, bicycling, gardening, swimming, dancing, or everyday chores like vacuuming, 2 days per week: Of muscle-strengthening activity, such as lifting weights. You can also try to exercise most days of the week, and even small amounts of physical activity can add up to give your health benefits.

h. Monitor Blood Sugar Levels: If you're at risk for diabetes or have prediabetes, monitoring your blood sugar levels can help detect early signs and prompt action.

i. Manage Stress: Chronic stress can contribute to insulin resistance. Practice stress management techniques such as mindfulness, yoga, or hobbies that promote relaxation.

j. Realize when it is causing you a problem. You need to

make the connection between feeling tired or ill, with the pressures you are faced with. Don't ignore physical warnings such as tense muscles, over-tiredness, headaches, or migraines.

k.   Identify the causes. Try to identify the underlying causes. Group the possible reasons for your stress into those with a practical solution, those that will get better anyway, given time, and those you can't do anything about. Try to let go of those in the second and third groups – there's no point in worrying about things you can't change or things that will sort themselves out.

l.   Review your lifestyle. Are you taking on too much? Are there things you are doing which could be handed over to someone else? Can you do things in a more leisurely way? You may need to prioritize things you are trying to achieve and reorganize your life so that you are not trying to do everything at once.

m.   Stress kills, but you don't have to be a victim.

n.   Quit Smoking: Smoking increases the risk of developing diabetes and cardiovascular complications. Seek support to quit smoking if you currently smoke.

o.   Limit Alcohol Consumption: Excessive alcohol intake can lead to weight gain and increase blood sugar levels. Drink in moderation, if at all.

p.   Get Regular Check-Ups: Routine medical check-ups can

help detect diabetes or prediabetes early. Work with your healthcare provider to develop a personalized prevention plan. This is critical. Early detection is lifesaving. Don't wait until you are feeling sick. Go get regular check-ups.

MANAGING DIABETES EFFECTIVELY

For those already living with diabetes, effective management is essential to prevent complications and maintain overall health. Here are key strategies for managing diabetes:

Monitor Blood Sugar Levels: Regular monitoring helps you understand how your body responds to food, physical activity, medications, and other factors. Keep a log and discuss trends with your healthcare team.

Adopt a Healthy Eating Plan: Work with a registered dietitian to develop a meal plan that fits your lifestyle and medication regimen. Consistency in carbohydrate intake and meal timing can help stabilize blood sugar levels.

Stay Active: Physical activity remains crucial for managing diabetes. Choose activities you enjoy and aim for a combination of aerobic exercises (like walking or swimming) and strength training.

Take Medications as Prescribed: If you require

medications to manage diabetes, take them consistently as prescribed by your healthcare provider. Follow up regularly to adjust treatment plans if necessary.

Managing Stress and Mental Health: Diabetes management can be stressful. Prioritize self-care, relaxation techniques, and seek support from loved ones or a counselor if needed.

Stay Informed: Educate yourself about diabetes management, new treatment options, and lifestyle changes that can benefit your health. Attending educational workshops or support groups.

Prevent Complications: Regular screenings for eye, kidney, and cardiovascular complications are crucial. Take proactive steps to address any issues that may arise.

Engage with Support Networks: Connect with others living with diabetes through support groups or online communities. Sharing experiences and tips can provide valuable support and encouragement.

INSPIRING HOPE AND EMPOWERMENT

My journey with diabetes has taught me that while the challenges are significant, so too are the opportunities for resilience and growth. By adopting a proactive approach to health, embracing the eight key health principles, and staying informed and engaged, individuals can empower themselves to live well with diabetes.

Each step you take towards better managing your health is a victory. Remember, you are not alone in this journey. Together, we can advocate for better healthcare access, promote wellness initiatives, and inspire hope in others facing similar challenges.

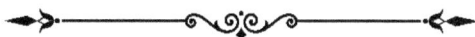

Reflection Question:

Reflect on one lifestyle change you can make today to reduce your risk of diabetes or better manage your current condition. How can you incorporate this change into your daily routine?

Practical Application:

Take a proactive step towards improving your health today. Whether it's scheduling a medical check-up, starting a new exercise routine, or making healthier food choices, commit to action. Track your progress and celebrate each milestone along the way.

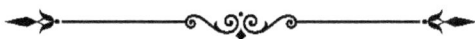

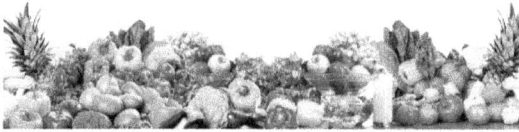

CONCLUSION

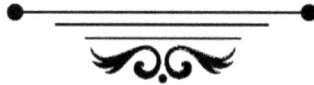

In closing, managing diabetes requires dedication, knowledge, and a willingness to adapt. Through my journey and the principles outlined, I hope to inspire and empower individuals to take charge of their health, reduce their risk of diabetes, and live a fulfilling life. Together, we can build a future where health disparities diminish, and hope for better outcomes flourishes.

Living with diabetes is undoubtedly challenging, but it is not insurmountable. Through my journey, I discovered that with the right approach and mindset, it is possible to manage, control, and even prevent the condition. I hope that by sharing my story and these eight key health principles, I can inspire and empower others to take control of their health and live a fulfilling life.

May your journey towards wellness be guided by resilience, compassion, and a commitment to living your best life. Here's to a healthier, brighter future for all. Remember, wellness is a matter of the mind, body and the heart.

REFERENCES

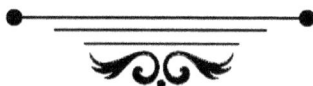

1. Centers for Disease Control and Prevention (CDC)
   https://www.cdc.gov/diabetes/php/data-research/index.html

2. https://minorityhealth.hhs.gov/diabetes-and-african-americans

3. https://www.pewresearch.org/science/2022/04/07/black-americans-views-about-health-disparities-experiences-with-health-care/

4. https://www.cdc.gov/diabetes/php/data-research/index.html

5. https://www.news-medical.net/health/Proactive-Health-The-Shift-Towards-Preventative-Healthcare.aspx

6. https://doihaveprediabetes.org/

7. https://www.niddk.nih.gov/health-information/diabetes/overview/preventing-problems/heart-disease-stroke

8. Barnard, Reversing Diabetes, 2007

9. https://www.verywellhealth.com/diabetes-and-heart-disease-risk-in-black-people-5222428

10. https://www.ncbi.nlm.nih.gov/pmc/articles/PMC420443
    1/

11. https://health.ucdavis.edu/blog/cultivating-health/3-
    ways-getting-outside-into-nature-helps-improve-your-
    health/2023/05

12. https://www.health.harvard.edu/staying-healthy/how-
    much-water-should-you-drink

13. https://www.webmd.com/a-to-z-guides/ss/slideshow-
    sunlight-health-effects

14. https://health.gov/myhealthfinder/healthy-living/mental-
    health-and-relationships/get-enough-sleep

15. President - Neal Barnard, MD, FACC (pcrm.org)

16. https://www.cdc.gov/healthy-weight-growth/physical-
    activity/index.html

17. Diabetes and African Americans:
    https://www.cdc.gov/diabetes/library/features/diabetes-
    and-african-americans.html

18. Heart Disease Facts:
    https://www.cdc.gov/heartdisease/facts.htm

19. Heart Disease and African Americans:
    https://www.heart.org/en/health-topics/consumer-
    healthcare/heart-disease-and-stroke-in-african-americans

20. NIH National Institute of Diabetes and Digestive and
    Kidney Diseases: https://www.niddk.nih.gov/

21. National Heart, Lung, and Blood Institute:
https://www.nhlbi.nih.gov/

22. Diabetes and African Americans:
https://www.diabetes.org/resources/statistics/statistics-by-topic/diabetes-and-african-americans

23. Journal Articles and Research Papers

24. Diabetes Care:
https://care.diabetesjournals.org/Circulation:
https://www.ahajournals.org/journal/circulation

25. Journal of the American College of Cardiology:
https://www.jacc.org/